Wu Qin Xi

in the same series

Ba Duan Jin
Eight-Section Qigong Exercises
Compiled by the Chinese Health Qigong Association
978 1 84819 005 4

Liu Zi Jue
Six Sounds Approach to Qigong Breathing Exercises
Compiled by the Chinese Health Qigong Association
978 1 84819 006 1

Yi Jin Jing
Tendon–Muscle Strengthening Qigong Exercises
Compiled by the Chinese Health Qigong Association
978 1 84819 008 5

Chinese Health Qigong

Wu Qin Xi

Five-Animal Qigong Exercises

Compiled by the Chinese Health Qigong Association

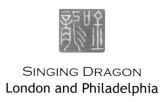

SINGING DRAGON
London and Philadelphia

First published in the United Kingdom in 2008 by
Singing Dragon
An imprint of Jessica Kingsley Publishers
116 Pentonville Road
London N1 9JB, UK
and
400 Market Street, Suite 400
Philadelphia, PA 19106, USA

www.jkp.com

First published in China in 2007 by Foreign Languages Press
24 Baiwanzhuang Road, Beijing, China
Copyright © Foreign Languages Press 2007

Library of Congress Cataloging in Publication Data
A CIP catalog record for this book is available from the Library of Congress

British Library Cataloguing in Publication Data
A CIP catalogue record for this book is available from the British Library

ISBN 978 1 84310 007 8

Disclaimer
This book is for reference and informational purposes only and is in no way intended as medical counseling or medical advice. The information contained herein should not be used to treat, diagnose or prevent any disease or medical condition without the advice of a competent medical professional. The activities, physical or otherwise, described herein for informational purposes, may be too strenuous or dangerous for some people and the reader should consult a physician before engaging in them. The author and Singing Dragon shall have neither liability nor responsibility to any person or entity with respect to any loss, damage, or injury caused or alleged to be caused directly or indirectly by the information contained in this book.

Printed and bound by
Reliance Printing (shenzhen)., Ltd, Hong Kong

Contents

Chapter I   Origins and Development   9

Chapter II   Characteristics   15

Chapter III   Practice Tips   21

Chapter IV   Step-by-Step Descriptions of the Routines . .   27

Section 1 Hand Forms, Stances and Maintenance of
Balance   28

Basic Hand Forms   28

Basic Stances   30

Maintenance of Balance   32

Section 2 The Exercises Illustrated   33

Ready Position: Adjusting the Breath   33

Tiger Exercise (虎戏)   37

Deer Exercise (鹿戏)   50

Bear Exercise (熊戏)   63

Monkey Exercise (猿戏)   75

Bird Exercise (鸟戏)   88

Winding-Down Exercise to Convey Qi to Dantian . . . 100

APPENDIX: ACUPUNCTURE POINTS
MENTIONED IN THIS BOOK 105

Preface

Wu Qin Xi or Five-Animal Exercises imitating the movements of animals and birds, is a group of physical and breathing exercises for health care with a uniquely Chinese national flavor. The system was designed by Hua Tuo, a leading physician of the Eastern Han Dynasty (25–220 AD). He developed his system based on existing ancient Chinese traditional physical exercises following theories of the functions of the internal organs and meridians as well as the principles of the circulation of Qi and blood in the human body. His inspiration came from careful observation and study of the characteristic behavior and activities of tigers, deer, bears, monkeys and birds. He came to the conclusion that wild creatures regularly performed certain exercises to build up their constitution and improve their life skills. This book *Wu Qin Xi* in the *Chinese Qigong Exercise Series* was edited by the Chinese Health Qigong Association. In this book, the physical movements and spiritual expressions of those creatures are vividly described, and the principles of traditional Qigong exercises are used as guidance for students. During practice of the exercises, they are asked to coordinate their mind with the movements, and combine internal exercises with external exercises. Wu Qin Xi is not designed just for superficial imitation of the outer attitudes of those animals, because this may discourage the students, diminish their enthusiasm and reduce the efficiency of practice. The postures and movements of the exercises are elegant, so as to stimulate enthusiasm for learning and practicing the exercises. The movements are comparatively simple, and easy to remember. They are also very safe, as the physical exertion required will not tax even older people. The technical requirements are not very complicated, and so they are not difficult to master, and can be undertaken by people of different age groups and degrees of experience.

Experience has proved that after a certain period of practice, both physical and mental health are improved. Indeed, physical and psychological tests of people who practice Wu Qin Xi give high scores to their overall constitution, the functions of the various organs, mental attitude and power of perception, as well as physical fitness. In addition, the waistline and ratio between waist and buttocks in female practitioners are reduced, the cardiovascular and respiratory functions are markedly improved, and the grip strength is reinforced. Subjective appraisal of the effectiveness of these exercises by practitioners has found enhancement of bodily strength, improvement of flexibility of joints, and enhancement of spiritual vitality and psychological confidence.

Chapter I

Origins and Development

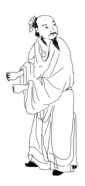

According to the Five-Animal Exercises can be traced back to remote *Lu's Chronicle* (呂氏春秋), Wu Qin Xi or the Five-Animal Exercises can be traced back to remote antiquity, as a treatment for swollen legs. A type of "dance" was devised for this purpose, which can be regarded as the embryo of the physical and breathing exercises developed in later ages in China. In *Zhuang Zi* (庄子), we find, "Exhaling to get rid of waste and inhaling fresh air, imitating the gait of a bear and the way a bird spreads its wings will prolong the life span." This is the earliest reference to the idea of health care by imitating the movements of wild creatures. In 1973, a wall painting titled, *Diagrams of Physical and Breathing Exercises* was excavated from an ancient tomb at Mawangdui in Changsha, Hunan Province. It shows people adopting dragon, snipe, bear, monkey, cat, dog, crane, swallow, and even tiger and leopard postures. This is clear, although some captions are difficult to read.

The formation of Wu Qin Xi is first mentioned in the *Biography of Hua Tuo* in *History of the Three Kingdoms* (三国志•华陀传),

written by Chen Shou of the Western Jin Dynasty (265–316). In this book, the author writes, "Hua Tuo developed a set of exercises called Wu Qin Xi, namely, first tiger, second deer, third bear, fourth monkey and fifth bird, as physical and breathing exercises to cure diseases and strengthen the feet for walking." In the Southern and Northern Dynasties period (420–589), Fan Ye, the author of the *Chronicle of the Later Han Dynasty* (后汉书), made a similar statement. Unfortunately, no illustrations or diagrams showing how to practice the original exercises as devised by Hua Tuo can be found in the ancient literature.

However, Tao Hongjing of the Southern and Northern Dynasties, in his *On Caring for the Health of the Mind and Prolonging the Life Span* (养性延命录), describes the exercises invented by Hua Tuo, and as he lived only about 300 years after the latter it is assumed that Tao's account is accurate. But as Tao Hongjing's explanations are not accompanied by illustrations, the exercises are difficult to practice. This deficiency is made up for somewhat in the Ming Dynasty (1368–1644) works, such as the *Marrow of the Red Phoenix* (赤凤髓) by Zhou Lüjing, and in the Qing Dynasty (1644–1911) works of the *Miraculous Book of Longevity* (万寿仙书) by Cao Wuji and *Diagrammatic Illustrations for Practice of the Five-Animal Dance* (五禽舞功法图说) by Xi Xifan, where the practical movements of the exercises are described in detail, with diagrams and drawings. These movements are much modified from those in Tao Hongjing's work in that besides the physical movements, the mental attitudes, concentration, etc., are also described. In addition, physical exercises are integrated with the adjustment of the circulation of Qi and blood. These ancient books provide a key basis for more modern studies of the exercise.

Many schools of Wu Qin Xi have sprung up in modern times, with different modifications of the exercises. Some schools even name themselves after Hua Tuo. Nevertheless, they all adhere to the fundamental principles of imitating the movements of the five wild creatures and combining physical with mental exercises. And they all have the common aim of strengthening muscles and bones, promoting the circulation of Qi and blood, preventing and curing diseases, maintaining good health and prolonging the life span.

The practice of Wu Qin Xi can be divided into two types: One emphasizes the physical exercise of the trunk and limbs to strengthen the bodily constitution. This is called "external exercise." The other emphasizes mental exercises which are supposed to imitate the spiritual activities and expressions of animals, to stimulate mental activity, this is called "internal exercise." The former division can be further divided into two groups. Vigorous practice mainly for self-defense is called "Five-Animal Boxing," which can also be used for treating illness by means of pounding or massage. When performed gently and gracefully, with the aim of strengthening the body constitution and improving the spiritual mood, it is called "Five-Animal Dance."

The sequential arrangement of exercises in this book was drawn from the *History of the Three Kingdoms*, namely in the order of tiger, deer, bear, monkey and bird exercises, and each section contains the two variations mentioned in Tao Hongjing's work. In addition, a starting posture for preparatory adjustment of the breath and an ending posture for return of Qi to its origin are arranged before and after the complete set of exercises.

Wu Qin Xi is easy to practice, especially by middle-aged and older people, through integrating exercises of the body, mind and Qi. The basic materials of this book were selectively collected from ancient works on the subject, and enriched with contributions from the modern sciences of human kinematics and physical aesthetics, as well as the basic theories of the internal organs and meridians in traditional Chinese medicine.

The physical movements are designed to show the courage and robustness of the tiger, the serenity and poise of the deer, the steadiness and solidity of the bear, the nimbleness and dexterity of the monkey and the swiftness and grace of the bird. The external physical movements are at all times integrated with accompanying exercises of the mental faculties.

Chapter II
Characteristics

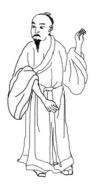

Symmetrical Movements, Safe and Easy to Learn

Wu Qin Xi is symmetrical and can be performed conveniently. One may perform either a complete set of exercises or a particular exercise repeatedly. They are safe aerobic exercises requiring only moderate physical exertion, and so practitioners may freely arrange the amplitude and intensity of physical exertion in accordance with their bodily constitution and strength.

The movements are rather simple, and both the dynamic and static exercises can be further divided into different parts and improved. For example, when "raising the tiger's paw" the movement of the hands can be divided into three stages, namely, pressing the palms downward, flexing the fingers and rotating the fists. The movement of the arms can be divided into four stages, namely, raising the arms to a horizontal level, raising them up further, pulling them back down to the original horizontal level and then pressing them downward. At the same time, the potential strength inside the body should be applied throughout the performance of the exercises, with the eyes following the hands' motion and the head bending forth and back accordingly. In the first stage of practice, concentrate on the physical movements. When these become natural and comfortable, proceed to the next stage, which involves combining the physical movements with the breathing exercises and the spiritual vivacity of the tiger.

Stretching the Trunk and the Limbs, and Flexing the Joints

Wu Qin Xi is an all-round set of movements, in which the trunk is turned to each side, bent in all directions, folded forward, backward, raised, lowered, contracted and expanded to exercise the spine. The waist is considered as the main axis of the body and the key linkage of the limbs. Therefore, exercising the limbs can further increase the movement range and amplitude of the spine, and improve the physical efficiency of the trunk.

Exercises of the fingers and toes are particularly emphasized for improving the blood circulation to the extremities. Also, as some groups of muscles are seldom used in daily life, special exercises have been designed to strengthen them, such as "antler clash," "running deer," "bear waist rotation," "monkey's paw" and "flying bird."

External and Internal Exercises
to Relax the Body and Concentrate the Mind

The ancients discovered that breathing exercises promote the circulation of Qi and blood, while physical exercises improve the functions of the joints, ligaments and muscles. Wu Qin Xi imitates the postures and movements of wild creatures. But it is important to keep in mind that the external physical activities are regulated by special mental activities. In the practice of Wu Qin Xi, you should imitate both the physical activities and the psychological character of the creature in question, i.e. the courage and robustness of the tiger, the calmness and serenity of the deer, the steadiness and solidity of the bear, the nimbleness and astuteness of the monkey, and the rapidity and grace of the bird. The external physical activities should follow and obey the internal will and thought. At the same time, the physical movements should be integrated with the breathing exercises, while concentrating on the given acupuncture point.

Students are advised to keep their muscles as relaxed as possible to ensure that the movements are performed comfortably and smoothly, while at the same time using the will to propel Qi and blood throughout the body.

Combining Dynamic with Static Exercises, and Integrating Physical Exertion with Mental Refreshment

In Wu Qin Xi, imitation of the postures and movements of wild creatures improves the flexibility of the body and limbs and the motility of the muscles and bones. At the same time, you should integrate the static exercises of the mind with the dynamic exercises of the body by the practice of so-called *"rujing"* (入靜), a mental exercise enabling you to "fall into a calm mood" by concentrating the mind on the physical activities and eliminating all mental distractions.

After completing the starting posture, closing posture and each movement, you should perform a pole-standing exercise to adjust the breath and keep yourself physically relaxed and mentally sedated for a while. Meanwhile, your mind enters a state of total empathy with the wild creatures, seeing in your mind's eye their alternating images and feeling the circulation of Qi in your body, so as to integrate physical relaxation with mental activity.

Therefore, alternating the two stages by adequately integrating dynamic and static exercises of both the body and the mind can produce a combined and mutually reinforcing effect.

Chapter III
Practice Tips

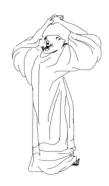

Requirements of the Body

The ancients held that "while exercising, if the body's posture is not correct, the breath, mind and spirit of the practitioner will all be disturbed." Before starting to exercise, the body should be held in a natural posture, with the head and back erect, chest slightly concave, shoulders relaxed and all the muscles relaxed. At the same time, you should calm your mind and breathe in a regular way. During exercise, the relevant animal's posture must be imitated as closely as possible. Pay attention to the starting and closing postures, practice each movement at the correct level, strength, speed and exactness, without any stiffness or sluggishness. Moderate and nimble physical exercise of the trunk and joints can slow the aging process.

Requirements of the Spirit

An important requirement of the spirit in the course of exercise is the integration of the physical activities of the body with its spiritual condition. During exercise, the spirit is the foundation for adjusting and supporting the physical activities of the body. A special characteristic of the spirit is its romantic charm, or "amusement." Different from other physical exercises, Wu Qin Xi should be practiced in a light-hearted manner, because a close imitation of the spiritual expressions of animals gives pleasure to the practitioners. When performing the tiger exercise, you should try to display the brave and wild temperament of the tiger, and in the deer exercise, adopt the rapid, smart and brisk pace of a trotting deer. While doing the bear exercise, imitate the heavy and steady walk of a bear in the forest; in the monkey exercise, try to imagine the nimble movements of a monkey climbing a tree; and in the bird exercise, imitate the posture of a crane with its beak raised.

Requirements of the Mind

The Yellow Emperor's Canon of Internal Medicine (黄帝內经)contains the following admonition: "The heart [i.e. the brain] is the commander-in-chief of all the internal organs. So any minor fluctuation of the heart may cause remarkable disturbances in the other organs." Mental activities and emotional disturbances certainly affect the functions of the internal organs. Therefore, in the practice of this exercise, you should strive for a good mental state, and eliminate any emotion or thought harmful to body health. A good way of doing this is, before starting to practice, to concentrate your attention on the Dantian (about two inches below the navel), and banish all mental distractions. During practice, try to identify with the mental mood of the relevant animal in preparation for imitating its physical activities. When practicing the tiger exercise, try to imagine yourself as a fierce tiger in the mountains about to pounce on its prey; in the deer exercise, imagine that you are about to lock horns with another deer on a green field; in the bear exercise, you are a bear roaming the forest, with its body swaying to and fro; in the monkey exercise, you become a monkey scrambling up a peach tree to pick its fruit; and in the bird exercise, you are a white crane on a river bank stretching its legs and spreading its wings, ready to fly away. The exercises of the body, mind and breath should be arranged and performed in an integrated way, to relieve blockages in the meridians and promote the circulation of Qi and blood through them.

Requirements of the Breath

You should constantly adjust your breathing according to intensity of the physical exertion you are undertaking and the physical condition of your body. Beginners should first learn how to perform each physical exercise correctly and comfortably. Only when you can perform the exercises with a relaxed body and calm mind should you begin to pay attention to adjusting your breathing. The ancients held that "people can be exhausted by over-ventilated breath and even injured by purposely held breath." So it is essential that you should avoid such abnormal breathing while exercising. When practicing Wu Qin Xi, try to coordinate your breathing with the physical exercises: Inhale when making upward movements to raise the limbs or stretch them outward, and exhale during movements to lower the limbs or draw them inward. Inhalation can also be done at the stage preparatory to a movement, and exhalation when a movement is about to be completed. In general, natural abdominal breathing with the buttocks taut is recommended. The breath must be natural, free and smooth, and not held or interrupted. The depth of breath and amount of air inhaled must be adequate, neither too much nor too little. When you have learned to coordinate physical exercises and breathing exercises you may gradually take increasingly slower and deeper breaths, with the passage of less air.

Learning the Exercises Step by Step

Although the starting and closing postures and 10 movements of Wu Qin Xi are simple and easy to learn, a long period of steady practice is necessary to make the performance skillful and elegant. Therefore, at the early stage it is recommended that you follow a teacher to do simultaneous exercises with a group to learn the change of posture and sequence of movements in each exercise. The movements of the upper and lower limbs may be separately learned and practiced, then the body trunk is used as a main axis to connect all the limbs together for complete exercise of the whole body. After each movement can be proficiently performed, the various movements of an exercise should be done in sequence. At the same time, you should try to gradually combine breathing exercises with the physical exercises, and pay more attention to displaying the spiritual manner and mental mood of the relevant animal. This latter should be left to the final stage of your learning process. Wu Qin Xi must be learned and practiced step by step from the lower to the higher level, and from simple to complicated techniques. It is very important to lay a good technical foundation to avoid any harmful side effects.

Requirements of the Individual

Keep in mind your own bodily constitution when practicing Wu Qin Xi. This is especially important for middle-aged and older people, as well as people in poor health. The speed of the actions, height to which the limbs are raised, range of movement of the body and limbs, duration and frequency of practice, and intensity of physical exertion must be tailored to the individual. In general, an amount of exercise that makes you feel comfortable and pleasant is ideal. Some muscle soreness may be experienced, but the exercises should never be performed at such an intensity that the result is interference in one's normal daily life and work. Throwing oneself recklessly into the exercises can be harmful.

Chapter IV

Step-by-Step Descriptions of the Routines

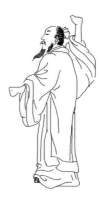

Section 1

Hand Forms, Stances
and Maintenance of Balance

Basic Hand Forms

Tiger's paw

Spread the fingers. The space between the thumb and the index finger is especially wide. The first and
second digital joints are bent inward (Fig. 1).

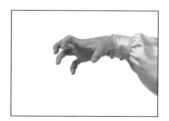

Fig. 1

Deer's antler

The thumb is extended and abducted, the index and little fingers are extended, and the middle and ring fingers are flexed (Fig. 2).

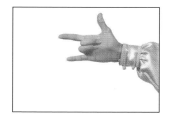

Fig. 2

Bear's paw

Connect the tips of the thumb and index finger to make a circle, with the other fingers flexed to make a hollow fist (Fig. 3).

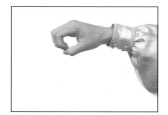

Fig. 3

Monkey's hooked paw

Connect the tips of the fingers and thumb, with the wrist flexed (Fig. 4).

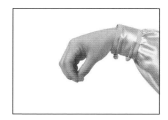

Fig. 4

The fingers and thumb are extended, the thumb, index and little fingers are tilted upwards, and the middle and ring fingers are juxtaposed downwards (Fig. 5).

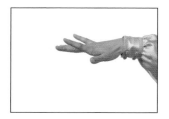

Fig. 5

Solid fist

Wi th the t ip of the thumb pressing the palm end of the ring finger, the other four fingers are folded over the thumb to make a solid fist (Fig. 6).

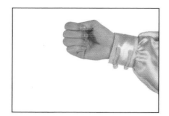

Fig. 6

Basic Stances

30

Bow stance

Stand with one leg in front of the other, separated by one large step and transversely at an adequate distance. The front leg is bent like a bow, with the knee directly above the tips of the toes, which are turned slightly inward. The rear leg is extended naturally, with the foot flat on the ground and its toes turned slightly inward (Fig. 7).

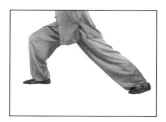

Fig. 7

Empty stance

Move one foot forward one step. Rest the heel lightly on the ground, with the toes tilted upward and the knee slightly flexed; the rear knee is bent in a preliminary squat position; the sole of the rear foot is squarely on the ground with its tip pointing more forward than laterally; the hip is just above the heel of the rear foot to support the body weight (Fig. 8).

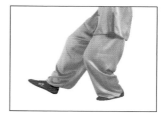

Fig. 8

T-stance

With the feet 10–20 cm apart, both knees are bent, with the heel of one foot lifted up and the tip of the toes just touching ground beside the arch of the other foot; the body descends to a semi-squat position; the sole of the other foot is placed squarely on the ground to support the body weight (Fig. 9).

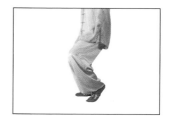

Fig. 9

Maintenance of Balance

Stand straight on one leg with the upper body erect; raise the other knee, with the shin perpendicular and the toes pointing downward (Fig. 10).

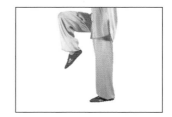

Fig. 10

Stand upright on one leg, with the other extended straight backward and raised from the ground, foot pointed in line with the leg and the toes pointing downward (Fig. 11).

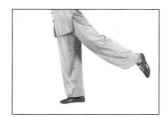

32

Fig. 11

Section 2

The Exercises Illustrated

Ready Position: Adjusting the Breath

First position: Stand with the feet close together, the arms hanging naturally at the sides of the thighs, the chest and abdomen relaxed. The head is kept erect, with the chin tilted slightly downward, the tongue touching the upper palate, and the eyes looking straight ahead (Fig. 12).

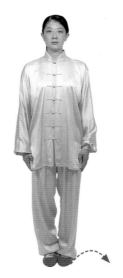

Fig. 12

Second position: The left leg moves one step to the left so that the feet are parallel and shoulder-width apart. Stand comfortably with both knees slightly bent. Take several deep breaths, and concentrate the mind on the Dantian some two inches below the navel (Fig. 13).

Third position: Bend the elbows and raise both arms upward to just in front of the chest, with the palms upward (Fig. 14).

Fourth position: Lower the arms, turn the palms inward and press them slowly down to the front of the abdomen. The eyes continue to look straight ahead (Fig. 15).

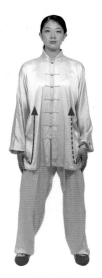 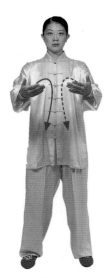 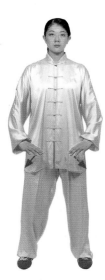

Fig. 13   Fig. 14   Fig. 15

Starting position: Repeat the third and fourth postures twice each, and let the arms hang loose once again (Fig. 16).

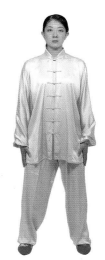

Fig. 16

☐ When raising and lowering the arms, do so gently and smoothly without pause, with the mind concentrated at the Laogong point (at the center of the palm between the second and third metacarpal bones—the point at which the tip of the middle finger reaches when making a fist).

☐ Inhale when raising the arms, and exhale when lowering them.

35

Common mistakes

☐ The body rocks while moving a foot to the left, with knees that are too straight.

☐ The palms are raised or lowered in a straight line, not in a curve, with the elbows laterally deviated and the shoulders shrugged.

☐ In order to maintain the balance, the knees should be slightly flexed, and the body weight settled on one foot before the other foot is lifted and moved. The foot should be moved slowly, landing on the ball of the foot.

☐ Before the arms are raised, concentrate on keeping the shoulders and elbows down, and allow the palms to move smoothly and naturally along an arc.

Functions and effects

☐ Eliminating mental distractions by assuming a quiet mood and adjusting the breath is a basic requirement for ensuring the optimum benefit from the exercises.

☐ Practice of the exercises helps to adjust the activity of Qi, promoting the ascent of clear Qi and descent of turbid Qi, and eliminating waste products and acquiring nutrients.

Tiger Exercise
(虎戏)

When performing the Tiger Exercise, exhibit the tiger's courage and fierceness, with the eyes glaring as if at the tiger's prey, and the hands stretched out and drawn back in powerful movements. The exercise should be done vigorously but with some softness from within—"as violently as a thunderstorm and as sedated and unshakably as Mount Tai."

Raising the tiger's paws (Routine 1)

First position: Let the arms hang loosely, with both palms turned to face the ground and the 10 fingers spread and flexed, like the paws of a tiger. Fix the eyes on the backs of the hands (Fig. 17).

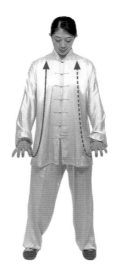

Second position: Turn the palms outward, flex the little finger first then

Fig. 17

the other four one by one to make fists, and raise the fists slowly along the front of the body to shoulder high (Fig. 18). Unclench the fists, and raise the hands as high as possible above the head. Then form the tiger's paws again. Fix the eyes on the backs of the hands (Fig. 19).

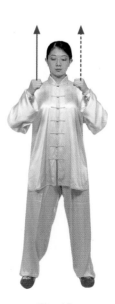

Fig. 18

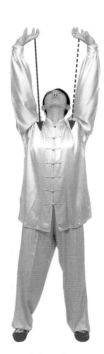

Fig. 19

Third position: Clench the fists once more, turning the palm sides to face each other. Keep the eyes fixed on the fists.

Fourth position: Lower the fists to shoulder level and unclench the fists (Fig. 20). Lower the hands with the palms down and the fingers extended to the front of the abdomen. Keep the eyes fixed on the backs of the hands (Fig. 21).

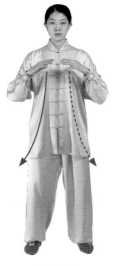

Fig. 20

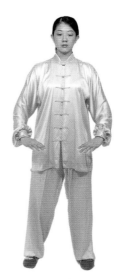

Fig. 21

Return to starting position

The first to the fourth positions are re-peated three times. Let the hands hang naturally at the sides of the thighs. Look straight ahead (Fig. 22).

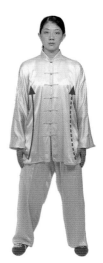

Fig. 22

Key points

- ☐ Concentrate the strength in the fingers as they are spread, bent to assume the tiger's paws, and turned outward to form fists.
- ☐ When raising the palms, throw out the chest and contract the abdomen to stretch the body, as if lifting a heavy weight. When lowering the palms, contract the chest and relax the abdomen to drive Qi into the Dantian.
- ☐ The eyes should always follow the movements of the hands.
- ☐ Inhale as the palms are raised, and exhale as they are lowered.

Common mistakes

- ☐ Failure to form a proper tiger's paw.
- ☐ Allowing the abdomen to protrude when raising the hands.

- To make a fist, first bend the first digital joint, then the second, and so on.
- When raising the hands above the head, keep the posture erect and immovable.

Functions and effects

- Clear air is inhaled when the palms are raised, and stale air is exhaled when they are lowered, so the circulation of Qi in Sanjiao (occupying the thoracic and abdominal cavities) is promoted and its functions adjusted.
- Forming a tiger's paw before making a fist reinforces the grip power and propels the blood circulation to the distal joints of the arm.

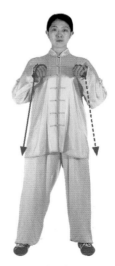

41

Seizing the prey (Routine 2)

First position: This exercise continues from the last position of the above exercise. Both fists, loosely clenched, are raised along the sides of the body to the front of the shoulders (Fig. 23).

Fig. 23

Second position: Both hands, with the fingers extended in tiger's paws and the palms facing down, are stretched straight out, and swung in an arc. At the same time, the upper body is bent forward with the chest thrown out, waist held tightly and eyes looking straight ahead (Fig. 24 front and side views).

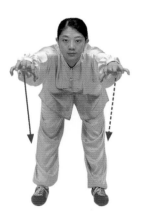

Fig. 24 front view

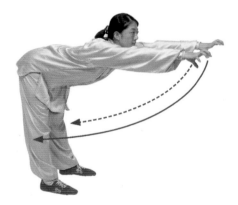

Fig. 24 side view

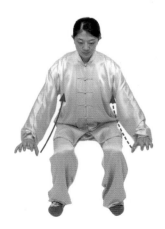

Fig. 25

Third position: Bend the knees, to assume a squatting position. Both chest and abdomen are contracted. Both hands, in tiger's paws, are moved in an arc line down to the outside of the knees, with the palms facing down. The eyes look ahead and down (Fig. 25). Then both knees are extended, the hips and abdomen move forward, and the upper body inclines backward. The hands, with hollow fists, are raised along the sides of the body to chest level. The eyes look straight ahead (Fig. 26 front and side views).

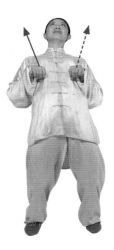

Fig. 26 front view

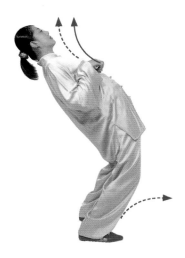

Fig. 26 side view

Fourth position: The left leg is lifted from the ground with the knee flexed and hands raised (Fig. 27).

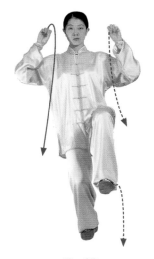

Fig. 27

Then it is moved forward one step to touch the ground with the heel. At the same time, the right knee is bent to lower the body to a squat position, to assume a left empty stance (no weight on the left foot), and the hands are changed into tiger paws and extended forward and downward to the outside of the knees with the palms facing down and the eyes looking downward—like a tiger pouncing on its prey (Fig. 28). Then the left leg is withdrawn, to assume the preparatory position (Fig. 29).

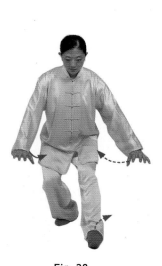

Fig. 28

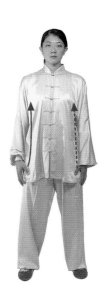

Fig. 29

Fifth to eighth positions: Repeat the first to the fourth positions, with the positions of the left and right sides of the body performed in reverse (Figs. 30–36).

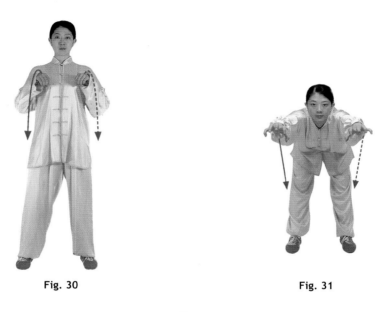

Fig. 30   Fig. 31

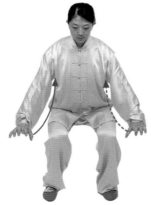

Fig. 32

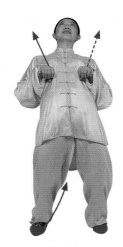

Fig. 33

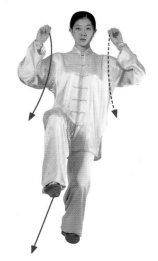

Fig. 34

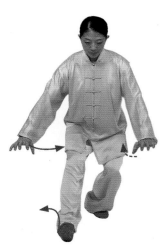

Fig. 35

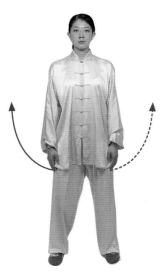

Fig. 36

Return to starting position: After the first to the eighth positions are completed, the palms are raised along the front of the body to the sides of the chest, with the palms facing up and the eyes looking straight ahead (Fig. 37). The elbows are then bent and the palms turned in and lowered to the sides (Fig. 38).

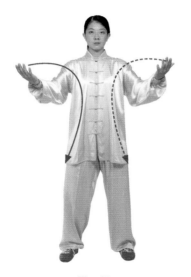

Fig. 33

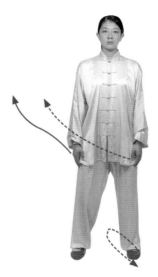

Fig. 34

Key points

☐ As the body is bent forward, both arms should be extended as far as possible, with the hips protruding backward and the spine fully extended.

☐ When the knees are flexed to allow the body to assume a squatting position, and the chest and abdomen are contracted, the extension of the knees, the thrusting forward of the hips and abdomen and the backward inclination of the body should be performed continuously and in coordination. The extension and flexion of the spinal column and the raising up and pressing down of the palms should also be performed in coordination.

□ The downward seizing of the prey position in the empty stance should be performed gently at first, and then more and more vigorously, accompanied by faster and deeper exhalation. The strength applied to perform the exercise is reinforced by Qi from Dantian, which should be extended to the finger tips, to show the braveness and fierceness of a tiger.

□ The vigor of the exercise and range of position should be reduced to suit the physical condition of older and weak people.

Common mistakes

□ Clumsy change of hand posture from fist to tiger's paw, and vice versa.

□ Insufficient extension of the body from the forward bending posture and lack of coordination between the hands and the body when the latter is extended.

□ Swaying of the body when adopting the empty stance.

Corrections

□ The seizing-the-prey exercise should be performed gently at first, and then more and more vigorously, concentrating the Qi as far as the finger tips. The withdrawal of the palms through an inwardly curving arc line should be performed vigorously at first, and then more and more gently, with the tiger's paw changed to a loose fist.

☐ As the flexed body is extended forward, both hands should be extended backward through an arc, to support the extension of the body.

☐ When stepping forward, keep the feet transversely apart to maintain the stability of the body.

| Functions and effects |

☐ The bending and extending exercises can improve the flexibility of the spine, increase the range of suppleness and flexion, and maintain the normal curvature of the spinal column.

☐ Exercise of the spinal column strengthens the lumbar muscles, helping to prevent and treat common problems of the waist, such as lumbar muscular strain and habitual strain of the waist.

☐ The Dumai meridian or governor vessel extends along the posterior midline (from Baozhong, an area in the lower abdomen upward to the Yinjiao point, near the upper gum) and the Renmai meridian or conception vessel extends along the anterior midline (from Baozhong upward to the Chengjiang point, to join the Dumai meridian at the Yinjiao point) of the body. Thus, bending and extending the spinal column can activate those meridians and remove blockages in them, promote the circulation of Qi and blood, and adjust the balance of Yin and Yang (the two opposing and interactive aspect of everything) in them.

Deer Exercise
(鹿戏)

Deer spring into a run, and suddenly stand still and alert for long periods of time. They wag their tails, and butt antlers with each other. Incorporating these movements, the practice of the deer exercise can activate the Dumai (governor vessel) and Renmai (conception vessel) meridians. The deer exercise should be performed lightly and gently. Extend your limbs with a comfortable and calm spirit, as if you were a deer playing freely and happily with other deer on the open plains and hillsides.

Colliding with the antlers
(Routine 3)

First position: The exercise is continuously performed from the last position of the previous exercise (the starting position). Both legs are slightly bent, with the body weight resting on the right leg. Step forward with the left foot past the inside of the right foot to the left front, with the heel touching the ground. At the same time, the body is slightly turned to the right. Make hollow fist with both palms and move them up to the level of the right shoulder with the bottom of the fists facing down and the eyes following the right fist (Fig. 39).

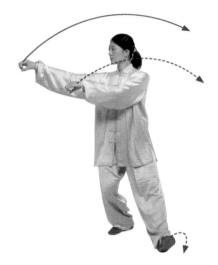

Fig. 39

Second position: The left leg is flexed, with the body weight shifted forward, and the left foot is placed firmly on the ground and turned outward. At the same time, the body is turned to the left, and both palms are moved upward and then to the left and backward through an arc after the "deer horn" posture is assumed by both hands with the palms facing outward and fingers pointing backward. The left arm is flexed, abducted and hotizontally extended, with the elbow touching the left side of the waist. The right arm is raised to the level of the forehead, and then extended backward to the left side, with the palm facing outward and the fingers pointing backward. The eyes should be fixed on the right heel (Fig. 40 front and side views).

51

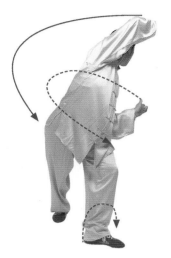

Fig. 40 front view

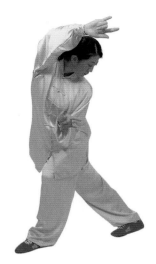

Fig. 40 side view

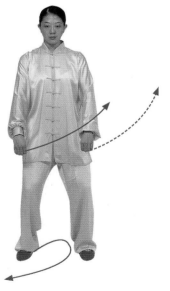

Fig. 41

Then the body is turned to the right side, and the left foot is withdrawn to stand with feet apart. At the same time, the hands are moved upward and then downward to the right in an arc and changed to hollow fists. Finally, they are dropped to hang at the sides, with the eyes looking straight ahead and downward (Fig. 41).

Third and fourth positions: The first two positions are repeated, reversing the positions of left and right Figs. 42–44).

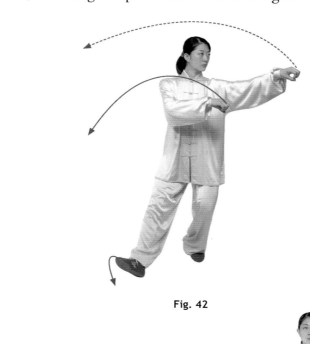

Fig. 42

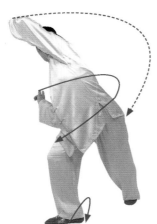

Fig. 43

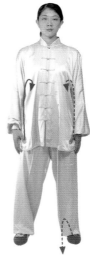

Fig. 44

Fifth to eighth positions: The same as the first four positions. After they are repeated, the eight positions are done once again.

Key points

- When the waist is rotated and bent laterally, the concave side of the waist should be stiff, while the convex side should be fully stretched by the backward extension of the raised arm.
- The posture of the lower limbs should be firmly maintained by fixing the heel of the rear foot stably on the ground to increase the rotating range of the abdomen and waist, just like a deer wagging its tail.
- The physical exercise should be combined with the breathing exercise: Inhale while raising the palms in an arc, and exhale while extending the palms backward.

Common mistakes

- Bending the body too far forward when the waist is rotated and laterally flexed.
- You cannot see your right heel, because the body is not laterally flexed enough.

- Keep the hips down with the force of the rear leg to maintain the erect posture of the upper body and increase the range of waist rotation.
- When shifting the body weight forward, flex the front knee more, and extend the raised arm further backward and downward.

Functions and effects

- The lateral flexion and rotation of the waist can fully turn the whole spine and reinforce the muscular strength of the waist to prevent and treat deposits of fat in the lumbar region.
- The exercise of lateral flexion and rotation of the waist with the eyes fixed on the rear heel can prevent and treat spinal problems.
- In the theory of traditional Chinese medicine, the waist is considered the house of the kidneys. Therefore, exercising the waist and hips can strengthen the waist, nourish the kidneys and improve the functions of the muscles and bones.

Running like a deer
(Routine 4)

First position: This exercise is continuously performed from the last position of the above exercise. The left leg is extended forward, with the knee flexed. At the same time, after both hands are changed to hollow fists they are moved upward and forward along an arc to shoulder level. The flexed wrists are shoulder-width apart, with the bottom of the fists facing down. Look straight ahead (Fig. 45).

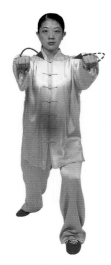

Fig. 45

Second position: Shift the body weight onto the back foot (the right in this case), and flex the right knee; stretch straight the left knee, keeping the sole of both feet flat on the ground. The neck and back are bent forward, with the abdomen contracted and the head facing down. At the same time, both arms are medially rotated and both hands are extended forward with the backs of the hands facing each other to assume a "deer antler" posture (Fig. 46 front and side views).

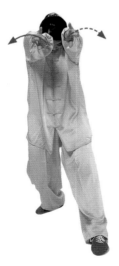

Fig. 46 front view

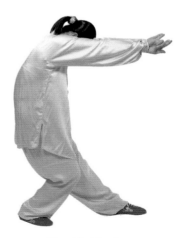

Fig. 46 side view

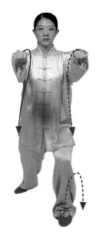

Fig. 47

Third position: The upper body is made erect, and the weight is shifted forward onto the left leg, with the left knee flexed and the right leg straightened to form a left bow stance. The shoulders are relaxed, the elbows down, the arms are laterally rotated, and the "deer antler" hands are changed to hollow fists with the backs of the hands uppermost and the eyes looking straight ahead (Fig. 47).

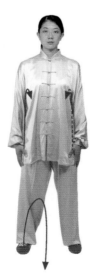

Fig. 48

Fourth position: The left foot is drawn back, to assume an open stance; fists are changed to palms and hang loosely at the sides. Look straight ahead (Fig. 48).

Fifth to eighth positions: The first four positions are repeated, with the left and right side actions reversed (Figs. 49–52).

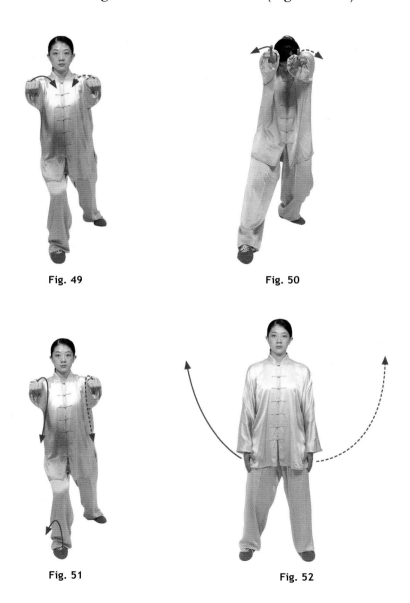

Fig. 49

Fig. 50

Fig. 51

Fig. 52

Return to starting position: After the eight positions are repeated once again, the hands are raised sideward up to shoulder height, with the palms facing up and the eyes looking straight ahead (Fig. 53). Both elbows are flexed and both palms are drawn close to each other, pressed downward and allowed to hang freely beside the body. The eyes continue to look straight ahead (Fig. 54).

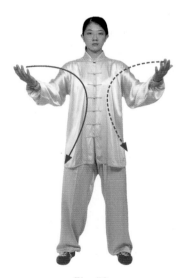

Fig. 53

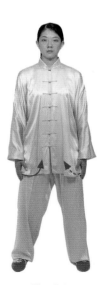

Fig. 54

- When moving one foot forward, move it in an upward arc and place it gently on the ground, to show the comfortable and calm spirit of a deer.
- When shifting the body weight backward, the arms should be extended forward, the chest contracted, the back flexed to assume a "horizontal bow-like" shape; then the head is protruded forward, the back protruded backward, the abdomen contracted and the hips held stiff to assume a "vertical bow-like" shape with the waist and back fully extended and stretched.
- Inhale when shifting the body's weight backward, and exhale when shifting it forward.

Common mistakes

- In the left bow stance, both feet are in a straight line, resulting in an unstable balance, so the upper body is distorted and difficult to relax.
- The "horizontal bow-like" shape of the back and the "vertical bow-like" shape of the trunk are not adequately performed.

61

Corrections

- An adequate transverse distance between the feet should be maintained when a step is made straight forward from the shoulder.

- The contraction of the chest can be increased by further medial rotation of the shoulders and upper arms. The backward protrusion of the trunk can be increased by increasing the forward protrusion of the head and hips, and the contraction of the abdomen.

Functions and effects

- The muscles of the shoulders and back can be stretched by medial rotation and forward extension of the arms to prevent and treat frozen shoulder and cervical syndrome. Assuming a bow-like back and contracted abdomen can reinforce the strength of the waist and back, to correct deformity of the spinal column.
- When stepping forward, the Dantian may be filled with Qi, and when shifting the weight backward, Mingmen (on the posterior middle line of the body and in the depression between the second and third lumbar spinal process) may be activated by Qi to communicate congenital Qi and postpartum Qi, and promote circulation of Qi through the Dumai meridian to activate the Yang Qi of the whole body.

Bear Exercise
(熊戏)

The natural manner marked by clumsiness, heaviness and slowness of a bear should be imitated when practicing the bear exercise. In the practice of this exercise, the circulation of Qi is guided by the mind to sink down to the Dantian (about two inches below the navel). The external exercise should be performed dynamically and vigorously, while the internal exercise should be performed stably and softly, to show the ponderousness and slow movements of a bear externally and at the same time to reflect the animal's keen intelligence internally.

Rotating the waist like a bear (Routine 5)

First position: This exercise is continuously performed from the last position of the above exercise (the starting position). Make hollow fists to imitate a bear's paws, the thumb sides facing each other, and hang them in front of the abdomen. Fix the eyes on the fists (Fig. 55).

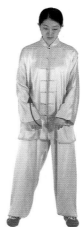

Fig. 55

Second position: The upper body is rotated clockwise, with the waist and abdomen as the axis. At the same time following the rotation of the body, both fists are moved along a circle over the right chest wall, upper abdomen, left chest wall and lower abdomen. The eyes should follow the rotation of the upper body (Figs. 56–59).

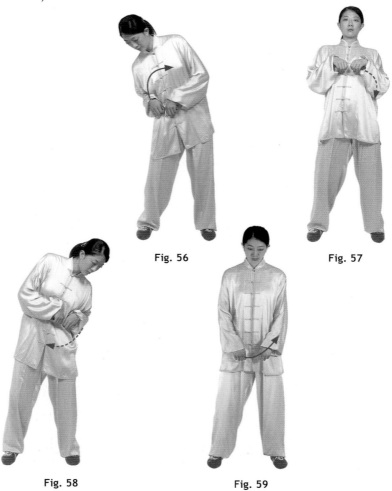

Fig. 56

Fig. 57

Fig. 58

Fig. 59

Third and fourth positions: Same as first and second positions.

Fifth to eighth positions: The first four positions are repeated, with the left and right sides reversed (Figs. 60–63).

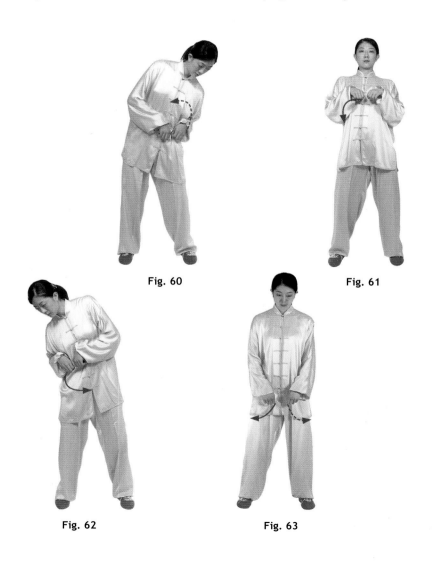

Fig. 60

Fig. 61

Fig. 62

Fig. 63

Return to starting position: After the last position has been completed, the fists are relaxed into palms and allowed to hang freely beside the body, with the eyes looking straight ahead (Fig. 64).

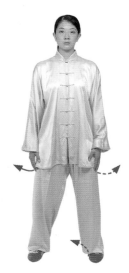

Fig. 64

| Key points |

- [ ] The hands should synchronize naturally with the rotation of the upper body.
- [ ] The movement of the hands is an external exercise, but the rotation of the waist and abdomen is driven by an internal force to promote the circulation of Qi in the abdomen to the Dantian. Inhale when lifting upward, and exhale when leaning forward and downward.

| Common mistakes |

- [ ] The hands are held too close to the abdomen or moved on their own instead of keeping in step with the rotation of the waist and abdomen.
- [ ] Exaggeration of rotation of the upper body.

□ Before starting the exercise, place both palms lightly on the waist and abdomen, with the shoulders and elbows relaxed, and let the rotation of the waist and abdomen drive the movement of the hand.

□ In this exercise, the waist and hips should be relatively fixed as the axis on which to rotate the upper body, with a feel of moving along a vertical circle. When the upper body is rotated upward, expand the chest and hold in the abdomen with waist and abdomen extended. When the body is rotated downward, try to constrict the chest and relax the abdomen, to apply pressure to the stomach, liver and spleen in upper abdomen.

Functions and effects

□ The exercise of the lumbar joints and muscles can prevent and treat lumbar muscular strain and soft tissue injury of the back.

□ Rotation of the upper body around the waist and abdomen, accompanied by the hands can promote the circulation of internal Qi and improve the functions of the stomach and spleen.

□ It can also produce a massaging effect on the digestive organs, to prevent and treat indigestion, poor appetite, abdominal distension and constipation.

Swaying like a bear
(Routine 6)

First position: This exercise is continuously performed from the last position of the above exercise. The weight is shifted onto the right leg, and the left foot is lifted from ground by raising the left hip and slightly flexing the left knee. Form hollow fists, with the eyes looking straight ahead (Fig. 65).

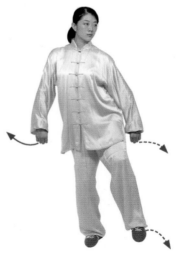

Fig. 65

Second position: The weight is shifted forward by straightening the right leg and moving the left foot to the left front side of the body with the sole placed flat on the ground and pointing forward. The body is turned to the right, the left arm is rotated outwards and extended forward, and the left fist is placed above and in front of the left knee with the palm facing left. The right fist is moved backward behind the body, with its palm facing backward, and the eyes looking straight ahead (Fig. 66).

Third position: The body is turned from the right side to the left side. The body weight is shifted backward by flexing the right knee and straightening the left leg. Rotate the waist and shoulders. The arms should describe an arc front and back. The right fist is placed above and in front of the left knee, with its palm side facing the right side. The left fist is moved backward behind the body, with its palm facing backward and the eyes fixed on the left front side (Fig. 67).

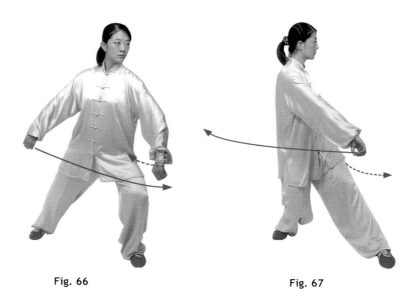

Fig. 66   Fig. 67

Fourth position: Turn the body from left to right, with the body weight shifted forward by flexing the left leg and extending the right leg. At the same time, the left arm is medially rotated and moved forward, with its fist placed above and in front of the left knee and the palm facing left. The right fist is moved backward behind the body, with its palm facing backward, and the eyes fixed on the left front side (Fig. 68).

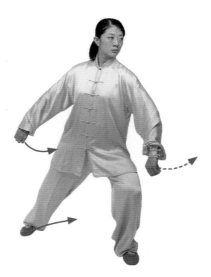

Fig. 68

Fifth to eighth positions: The first four positions are repeated, with the left and right sides reversed (Figs. 69–72).

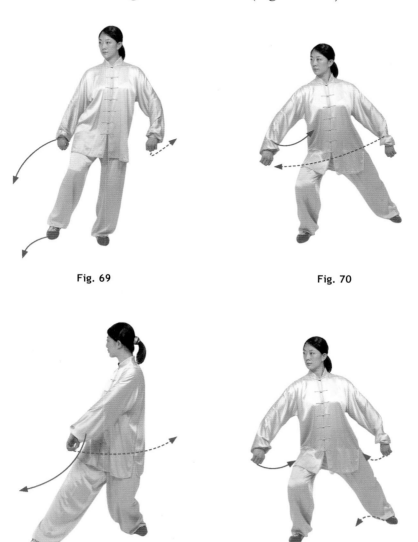

Fig. 69

Fig. 70

Fig. 71

Fig. 72

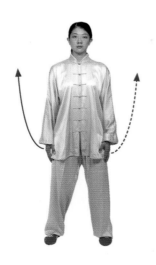

Fig. 73

Return to starting position: After the eight positions are repeated, the left foot is moved forward, to assume the starting position. At the same time, both hands are allowed to hang freely beside the body (Fig. 73). Both arms are raised to the lateral front of the body, at chest level, with the palms facing upward and the eyes looking straight ahead (Fig. 74). Both elbows are flexed, and the palms are rotated medially. The palms are then pressed downward and allowed to hang freely beside the body, with the eyes looking straight ahead (Fig. 75).

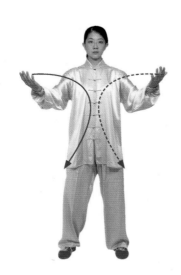

Fig. 74

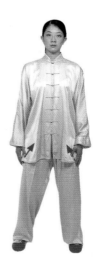

Fig. 75

- The thigh is raised by contracting the lateral group of lumbar muscles, then flexing the knee.
- When stepping forward, the foot is moved laterally at a distance wider than the width of the shoulders. Place the foot heavily on the ground to produce a tremor which is transmitted to the hip joint, imitating the heavy walk of a bear.

Common mistakes

- Raising the leg and flexing the knee without first lifting the hip.
- Placing the sole of the foot on the ground too lightly to produce a tremor, which should be transmitted to the hip joint.
- Corrections
- Practice lifting each hip in advance of the complete exercise: Keep the shoulders level when shifting body weight onto one leg and raising the other leg by first lifting the hip on the side, and vice versa.
- When placing the sole of the foot on the ground, the ankle and knee joints should be relaxed for transmission of the tremor to the hip joint.

73

Functions and effects

- The turning of the body to each side may affect the epigastric region so as to adjust the functions of the liver and spleen.

☐ Walking by lifting the hips and the shake produced by heavy stepping may reinforce the strength of muscles around the hip joint, maintain the body's balance and prevent and treat weakness of the lower limbs in older people, damage to the hip joint and pain in the knee joint.

Monkey Exercise
(猿戏)

The monkey is a clever and nimble animal, fond of scampering about and climbing trees. When performing the monkey exercise, try to imitate the light and swift movements of the monkey, but for the internal exercise you should keep your mind like a bright moon shining in the quiet and still night. So the monkey exercise is externally dynamic and internally static.

Lifting the monkey's paws (Routine 7)

First position: This exercise is continuously performed from the last position of the above exercise (the starting position). Both hands are placed in front of the body with the fingers extended and separated from each other (Fig. 76).

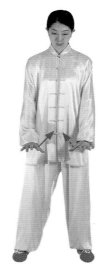

Fig. 76

Then the wrists are flexed and the fingers assembled to assume the hook-like paws of a monkey (Fig. 77).

Second position: The hands are lifted to chest level, with the shoulders shrugged, the abdomen contracted and the anus clenched. At the same time, the heels are lifted up and the head is turned to the left. The eyes look directly to the left (Fig. 78 front and side views).

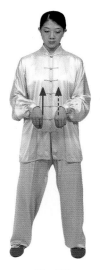 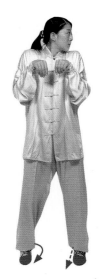 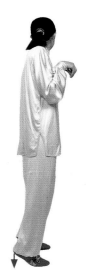

Fig. 77   Fig. 78 front view   Fig. 78 side view

Third position: The head is turned back to the front, the shoulders, abdomen and buttocks are relaxed, the heels are put back on the ground, and the hands are kept at shoulder level, wi th the f inge r s extended and palms facing down. The eyes look straight ahead (Fig. 79).

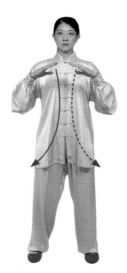

Fig. 79

Fourth position: The palms are pressed down and hang by the sides. The eyes look straight ahead (Fig. 80).

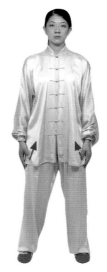

Fig. 80

Fifth to eighth positions: The first four positions are repeated again, but with the head turned to the right (Figs. 81–85).

Return to starting position: After the eight positions are repeated, the starting position is resumed.

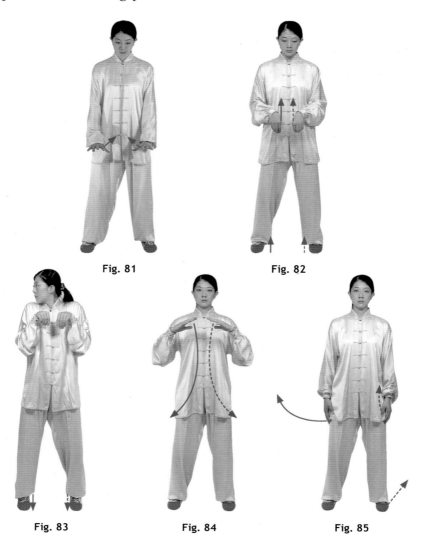

Fig. 81

Fig. 82

Fig. 83

Fig. 84

Fig. 85

- The assumption of the monkey's paw should be performed quickly.
- Shift the center of the body weight upward in the sequence of shrugging the shoulders, contracting the abdomen, tightening the anus, rising on the toes and then turning the head. All should be performed to the maximum degree.
- The physical exercise should be done in coordination with the breathing exercise: Inhale while lifting the hands and tightening the anus, and exhale while pressing the hands down, with the anus relaxed.

Common mistakes

- Wobbling when raising the heels is caused by faulty shifting of the body's weight.
- Inadequate shrugging of the shoulders and contraction of chest, back and upper limbs.

Corrections

- In order to maintain a stable stance, try to raise the top of your head exactly vertically, and smoothly shift your body weight.
- The whole upper body should be focused on a center at the middle point of the sternum, with neck, shoulders and arms closely assembled together, to imitate the physique of a monkey.

- □ The quick assumption of the monkey's paw can enhance the neuromuscular response.
- □ Lifting the hands while shrugging the shoulders, and contracting the chest to inhale can reduce the capacity of chest and compress the cervical blood vessels. Returning to the original posture may expand the chest capacity and that of the blood vessels, thereby improving the breathing, massaging the heart and improving the blood supply to the brain.
- □ Standing on the toes can reinforce the muscular strength of the legs and improve the balance.

Picking fruit (Routine 8)

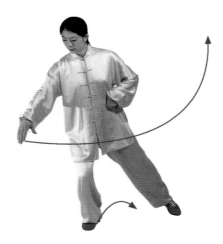

First position: This exercise is continuously performed from the last position of the above exercise. The left foot is moved to the left rear side with the tips of the toes touching the ground and the weight on the right leg. The right knee is flexed. Mean-

Fig. 86

while, the left elbow is flexed and the left hand assumes the monkey's paw at the left side of the waist. The right hand, palm facing down, is held at the front right side of the body (Fig. 86).

80

Second position: The weight is shifted backward, onto the left foot, which is placed solidly on the ground, with the left knee flexed to enable a squatting position. The right foot is withdrawn to the side of the left foot, with the tips of the toes touching the ground, forming a right T-stance. At the same time, the right palm is moved first downward over the abdomen and then upward to the left side in an arc, to just beside the face, with the palm facing the left temple. The eyes should follow the movement, and then the head should turn up to right front (Fig. 87).

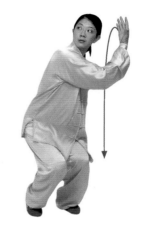

Fig. 87

Third position: The right hand is moved, palm down, along the left side of the body to the level of the left hip. The eyes should follow the hand's movement (Fig. 88). Move a big step with the right foot towards right front, straighten it and extend the left foot until only the tips of the toes are touching the ground,

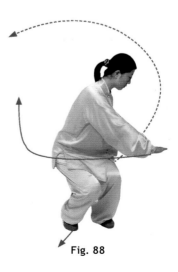

Fig. 88

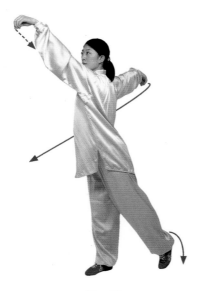

Fig. 89

shifting the body weight onto the right leg. Meanwhile, the right palm moves up in an arc past the front of the body to the right until it is slightly above shoulder height to assume a monkey's paw; while the left one moves forward and upward with the wrist flexed and the fingertips together as if plucking fruit from a tree. The eyes should be fixed on the left hand (Fig. 89).

Fourth position: The weight is shifted backward, the left hand forms a solid fist, and the right hand hangs loose at the front right side of the body, the thumb side facing the front (Fig. 90). The left knee is flexed and the right foot is drawn back to the side of the left foot, touching the ground with the toes to assume a right T-stance. At

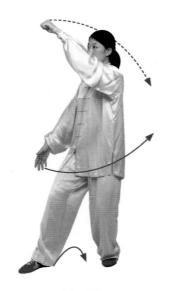

Fig. 90

the same time, the left elbow is flexed, and the left hand is drawn back to beside the left ear, with the palm facing upward and the fingers separated, as if holding a peach. The right palm is moved in an arc past the front of the body to just below the left elbow, to seemingly support it. Both eyes are fixed on the left palm (Fig. 91).

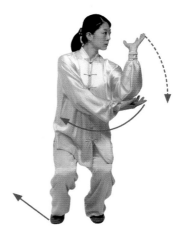

Fig. 91

Fifth to eighth positions: The first four positions are repeated, but the left and right positions are reversed (Figs. 92–97).

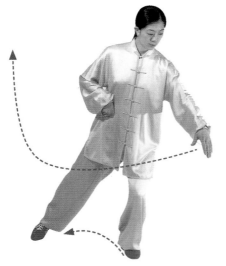

Fig. 92

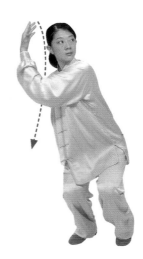

Fig. 93

83

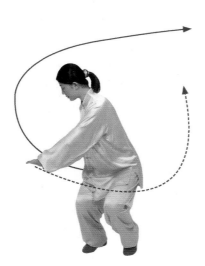
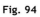

Fig. 94

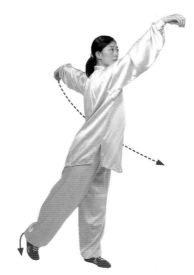

Fig. 95

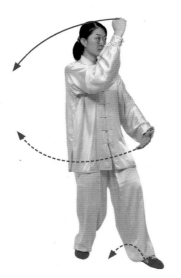

Fig. 96

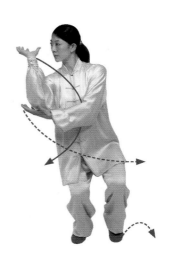

Fig. 97

Return to starting position:
After the eight positions are repeated, the starting position is resumed (Fig. 98). Both palms are raised to the front lateral sides at chest level, with the eyes looking straight ahead (Fig. 99). Both palms are moved close to each other, pressed downward with elbows bent, and allowed to hang loose at the sides, with the eyes looking straight ahead (Fig. 100).

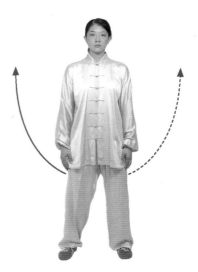

Fig. 98

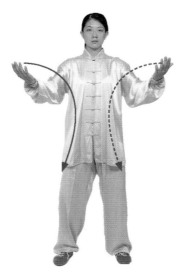

Fig. 99

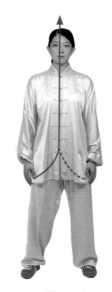

Fig. 100

- The eyes should follow the arm movements, imitating the sharp glances of a monkey.
- Contract the body when squatting down, but fully expand it when making a step forward, as if reaching for something above the head. The monkey fist should be formed quickly as if reaching for a peach, and opened quickly as if supporting a peach on the palm.
- Try to imitate the nimble and sudden movements of a monkey, but without too much exaggeration.

Common mistakes

- Lack of coordination between the exercises of the upper and lower limbs.
- When imitating picking a peach, the palm tends to move in a straight line rather than an arc, and the monkey's paw cannot be made in time.

Corrections

- When squatting down, the upper arm should be held close to the body, with the elbow flexed. When stepping forward, the arm should be fully stretched.
- When "picking a peach," the hand should be moved in an arc, and the monkey's paw should be made only when the hand reaches the proper position.

☐ The movement of the eyes accompanying the rotation of the neck can improve blood circulation in the brain.

☐ The complicated exercise of imitating a monkey picking a peach can integrate physical and mental activities, and alleviate pressure on the brain. Therefore, it is useful for preventing and treating nervousness and depression.

Bird Exercise
(鸟戏)

The bird exercise involves imitating a crane, traditionally regarded in China as a symbol of calmness, litheness, and longevity. In the practice of this exercise, you should imitate a crane standing upright, with its beak uplifted and displaying a carefree and contented mood, as well as the relaxed manner with which it flaps its wings. Protrude the neck and stiffen the back to drive the flow of Qi upward when raising your arms. Contract the chest and relax the abdomen to drive the flow of Qi downward to the Dantian in the lower abdomen when bringing your arms together downward. The bird exercise can promote circulation of Qi and blood in all the meridians and improve the motility of all the limbs.

Stretching upward
(Routine 9)

First position: This exercise is continuously performed from the last position of the previous exercise (the starting position). Adopt a semi-squatting position. With the palms facing downward and the fingers pointing forward, place one hand on top of

the other at the level of the abdomen.
The eyes should be fixed on the hands
(Fig. 101).

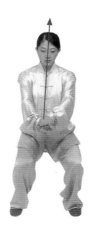

Fig. 101

Second position: Raise both hands above the head. The body is inclined slightly forward, with the shoulders shrugged, neck contracted, chest thrown out, waist protruded forward and eyes looking straight ahead (Fig. 102 front and side views).

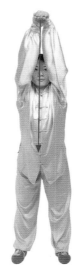

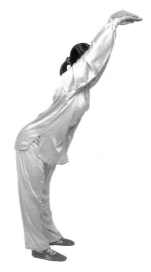

Fig. 102 front view   Fig. 102 side view

Third position: Adopt a semi-squatting position, with the hands and eyes as in the first position (Fig. 103).

Fourth position: The weight is shifted to the right side, the right leg is straightened, and the left leg is lifted from the ground and extended backward. At the same time, both arms are spread to the sides to imitate a bird's wings, with the palms facing up, chin, neck, chest and waist protruding, and eyes looking straight ahead (Fig. 104 front and side views).

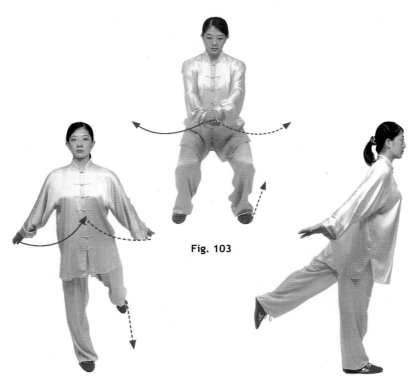

Fig. 103

Fig. 104 front view

Fig. 104 side view

Fifth to eighth positions: The first four positions are repeated, with the left and right sides reversed (Figs 105–108).

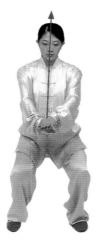

Fig. 105

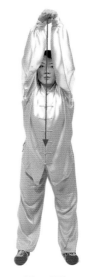

Fig. 106

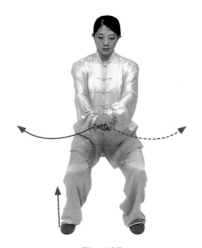

Fig. 107

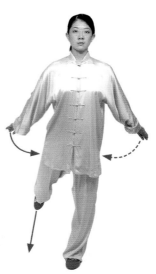

Fig. 108

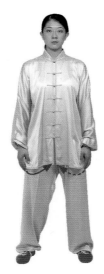

Fig. 109

Return to starting position: After the eight positions are repeated, the left foot is put back on the ground, with the feet apart, arms hanging loosely at the sides and the eyes looking straight ahead (Fig. 109).

Key points

- ☐ The overlapped hands should be placed at a convenient distance from the abdomen.
- ☐ Contract the neck, shoulders and hip region when raising the hands, and relax those parts of body when lowering the hands. The body should be protruded forward to assume a bow shape when the arms are extended backward.

Common mistakes

- ☐ Inadequate adjustment of the tightness and looseness of the body.
- ☐ Failure to maintain proper balance while standing on one leg.

- Before embarking on the exercise proper, practice overlapping the hands in front of the body, and contracting the body when the hands are raised and relaxing it when the hands are lowered.
- For maintenance of balance, shift the weight to the slightly flexed supporting leg before the other leg is extended backward. A straightened supporting leg helps to make the posture more stable.

Functions and effects

- By raising the hands, the chest capacity can be expanded, and the exhalation of waste air and flow of Qi to Dantian can be promoted by pressing the palms downward, improving the ventilation and vital capacity of the lungs. In addition, this movement can alleviate symptoms of chronic bronchitis and pulmonary emphysema.
- By raising the hands and extending the arms upward and backward, the Dumai and Renmai meridians can be stimulated.

93

Flying like a bird (Routine 10)

First position: This exercise is continuously performed from the last position of the above exercise. Adopt a semi-squatting stance, and allow the arms to hang in front of the abdomen with the palms facing each other. The eyes should look straight ahead and downward (Fig. 110).

Second position: The right leg is straightened, and the left leg is bent and lifted so that it forms a right angle, with the toes pointing down. At the same time, the arms are lifted together at the sides so that the hands, palms down, are located slightly higher than the shoulders. The eyes look straight ahead (Fig. 111).

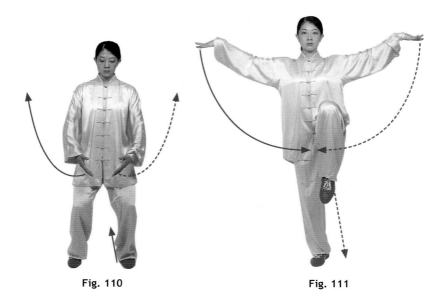

Fig. 110   Fig. 111

Third position: In a semi-squatting posture, place the tips of the toes of the left foot on the ground beside the right foot. At the same time, both hands are moved to the front of the abdomen with the palms facing each other. The eyes look straight ahead and down (Fig. 112).

Fourth position: Straighten the right leg, and lift the left leg to form a right angle, with the toes pointing down. At the same time, both hands are raised upward over the top of the head until their backs almost touch, with the finger tips pointing up. The eyes look straight ahead (Fig. 113).

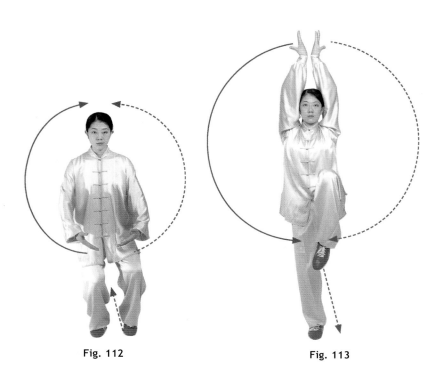

Fig. 112   Fig. 113

Fifth position: Land the left foot beside the right foot, the sole of both feet flat on the ground to assume a semisquatting posture, while returning the hands to their place in the first position. The eyes look straight ahead and down (Fig. 114).

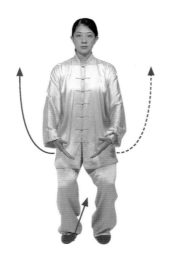

Fig. 114

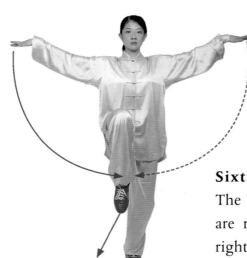

Fig. 115

Sixth to ninth positions: The second to fifth positions are repeated, but the left and right sides are reversed (Figs. 115–118).

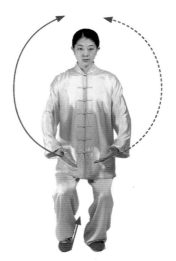

Fig. 116

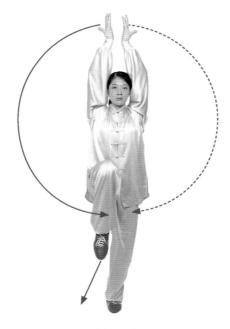

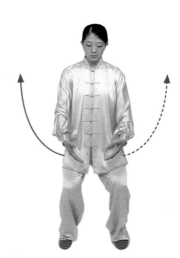

Fig. 117   Fig. 118

Return to starting position: After the second to ninth positions are repeated, both hands are lifted to the sides of the chest, with the palms facing up and the eyes looking straight ahead (Fig. 119). The elbows are flexed, and the palms are turned in and pressed down to hang loosely at the sides. The eyes look straight ahead (Fig. 120).

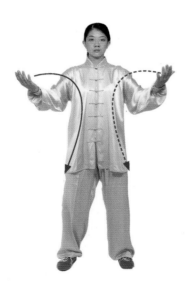

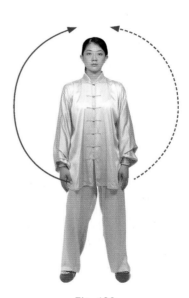

Fig. 119   **Fig. 120**

Key points

☐ When the arms are stretched out to the side, keep them as comfortably wide as you can, in order to expand the chest as much as possible. When they are moved to the centre of the body and downward, the chest should be contracted from both sides as much as possible.

☐ The upper and lower limbs should be moved in coordination and simultaneously.

☐ Inhale when raising the hands, and exhale when lowering them.

Common mistakes

☐ The arms are extended and moved in a stiff and ragged way.

☐ Shaky breathing and posture because of overtension.

Corrections

☐ The arms should be lifted up with a force conducted from the shoulders through a series of continuous wriggling positions, including first sinking the shoulders, then relaxing the elbows, and finally lifting the wrists. When lowering the arms, relax the shoulders first, then let the elbows drop down, and finally press palms down to the front of abdomen.

☐ When the arms are raised, inhale while raising the head as far as possible, chest thrown out and abdomen contracted. When lowering down the arms, exhale and relax the abdomen and waist, to promote flowing of Qi into the Dantian.

□ Combined with the breathing exercise, moving the arms up and down may promote respiration and expand the capacity of the chest, produce a massaging effect on the heart and lungs, and improve the blood's oxygenation function.

□ The upthrust of the thumb and index finger stimulates the Lung meridian (starting at the upper abdomen, extending along medial surface of the upper arms and stopping at the tips of the thumb and index finger), promotes circulation of Qi through this meridian, and improves the functions of the heart and lungs. Standing on one leg improves the sense of balance.

Winding-Down Exercise to Convey Qi to Dantian

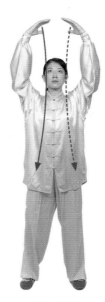

First position: Both hands are raised above the head, with the palms facing down (Fig. 121). Fig. 121

Fig. 121

Second position: Both palms are slowly pressed down to the front of the abdomen, with the fingertips pointing to each other and the eyes looking straight ahead (Fig. 122). This movement should be repeated once or twice.

Third position: The hands slowly describe a horizontal arc, navel high, as they approach each other with the palms facing each other and the eyes looking straight ahead (Fig. 123).

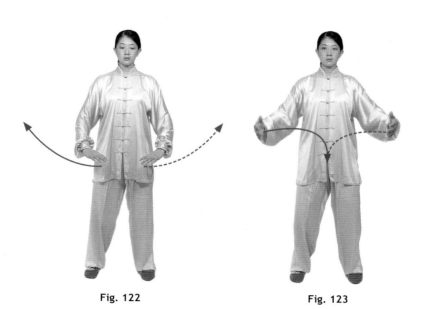

Fig. 122   Fig. 123

Fourth position: The hands are placed overlapping on the abdomen, the webs between the thumb and the index finger crossing each other. With the eyes half closed, calm the breath and concentrate the attention on the Dantian for a few minutes (Fig. 124).

Fifth position: Slowly open the eyes, and rub the palms together in front of the chest to produce a hot feeling in them (Fig. 125).

Sixth position: Rub the face all over with both palms three to five times (Fig. 126).

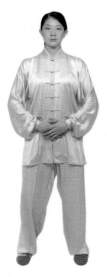
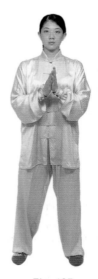
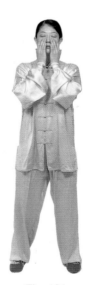

Fig. 124   Fig. 125   Fig. 126

Seventh position: Move the palms backward, rubbing the top of the head, the region behind the ears and down to the front of the chest, and then allow both arms to hang loosely beside the body. The eyes should look straight ahead (Fig. 127).

Eighth position: Move the left foot next to the right foot. Both feet should be flat on the ground, to resume the ready position, with the eyes looking straight ahead (Fig. 128).

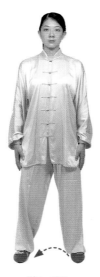

Fig. 127

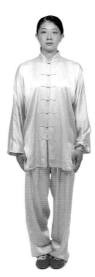

Fig. 128

| Key points |

- ☐ When pressing down the palms, the whole body should be relaxed from the head to the soles of the feet in succession.
- ☐ The hands should be moved naturally and smoothly when describing a horizontal arc in front of the navel, as if to collect

something from the front of the abdomen and convey it into the Dantian.

□ Involuntarily raising the chest and shoulders while raising the hands.
□ The hands fail to describe a proper arc.

Corrections

□ The body should be kept stable and well balanced and the shoulders relaxed when both arms are raised.
□ When the hands are raised along the sides of the body or describe an arc line in front of the abdomen, the mind should be concentrated at the center of the palms.

Functions and effects

104

□ "To conduct Qi back to its vessel" means to collect Qi acquired inside and outside the body in the course of physical exercise with smooth breathing, and convey Qi to the Dantian in order to keep the meridians in working order, regulate Qi and blood, and adjust the internal organs.
□ After rubbing the face with the palms, the body has been restored to its normal condition, and the exercise has been successfully performed.

Acupuncture Points
Mentioned in This Book

Baihui (GV20)

Taiyang (temple)

Yinjiao (GV28)

Chengjiang (CO24)

Dumai meridian (governor vessel)

Sanjiao meridian

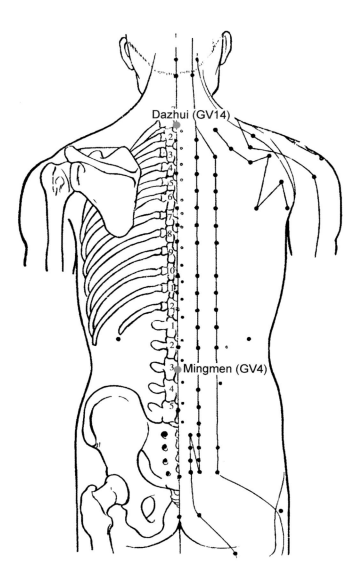

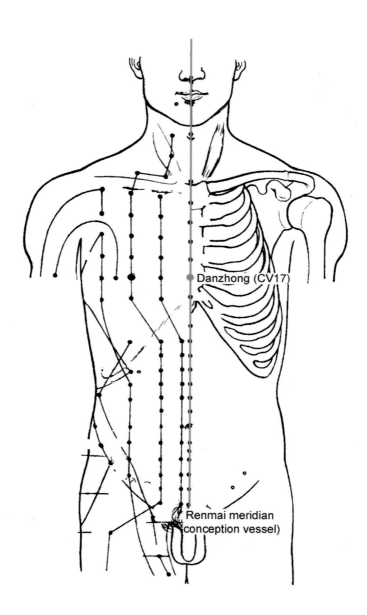

Danzhong (CV17)

Renmai meridian
(conception vessel)

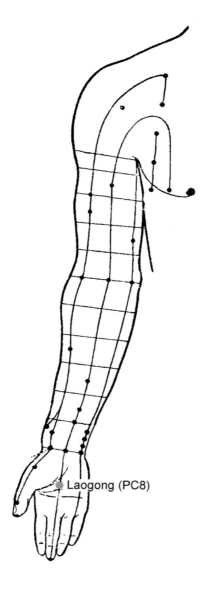

Laogong (PC8)

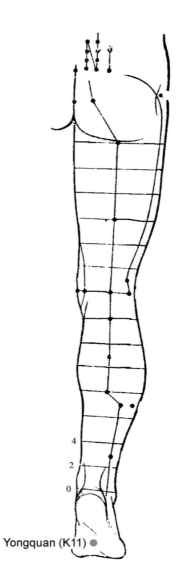

4

2

0

Yongquan (K11) ●